COSY KAMA SUTRA

HarperCollins*Publishers*
1 London Bridge Street
London SE1 9GF

www.harpercollins.co.uk

HarperCollins*Publishers*
Macken House, 39/40 Mayor Street Upper
Dublin 1, D01 C9W8, Ireland

First published by HarperCollins*Publishers* 2025

1 3 5 7 9 10 8 6 4 2

© HarperCollins*Publishers*, 2025
Illustrations of positions by Ollie Mann.
All other illustrations Shutterstock.com

Anna Mrowiec asserts the moral right to be identified
as the author of this work

A catalogue record of this book is available from the British Library

ISBN 978-0-00-880329-2

Printed and bound in the UK using 100% renewable electricity at
CPI Group (UK) Ltd

All rights reserved. No part of this publication may be reproduced,
stored in a retrieval system, or transmitted, in any form or by any
means, electronic, mechanical, photocopying, recording or otherwise,
without the prior written permission of the publishers.

Without limiting the exclusive rights of any author, contributor or the
publisher of this publication, any unauthorised use of this publication
to train generative artificial intelligence (AI) technologies is expressly
prohibited. HarperCollins also exercise their rights under Article 4(3)
of the Digital Single Market Directive 2019/790 and expressly reserve
this publication from the text and data mining exception.

This book is produced from FSC™ certified paper and other
controlled sources to ensure responsible forest management.

For more information visit: www.harpercollins.co.uk/green

COSY KAMA SUTRA

69 Positions for Maximum Pleasure and Minimum Draught

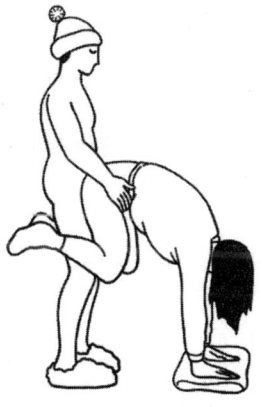

FANNY SNUGGLEBOTTOM

HarperCollins*Publishers*

Dedication

For my husband and human hot water bottle, James. You've inspired this book's contents and it would not exist without your regular, sustained input.

Disclaimer

The publisher and author recommend that all activities in *Cosy Kama Sutra* be undertaken with great care, pre-stretching and central heating. We accept no responsibility for injuries sustained during enthusiastic lovemaking, which may include (but are not limited to):

- light singeing from romantic candle arrangements or log-burning fireplaces
- overheating under several layers of fleece
- sudden-onset lactose intolerance due to excessive hot chocolate or fondue consumption
- genital chafing
- skin irritation or accidental entanglement in knitted garments
- and, in extreme cases, total and irreversible over-relaxation.

Please proceed with caution, hydration and easy access to a fire extinguisher.

INTRODUCTION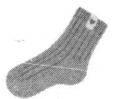

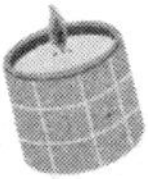

Welcome, reader and cosy erotica novice! I'm so glad you've picked up this book. You've taken the first step towards heating up your sex life – not too much, of course, but to a nice, tepid warmth that will spread through your body from your sexual organs to your toes.

This is the sex guide for those ready to choose comfiness over kinkiness, earmuffs over handcuffs, embers over fireworks – and would always welcome a post-coital mug of cocoa.

So snuggle up, strip down (a bit) and prepare to redefine *'Netflix and chill'*. Because nothing says romance like a shared weighted blanket and the faint scent of cinnamon lube.

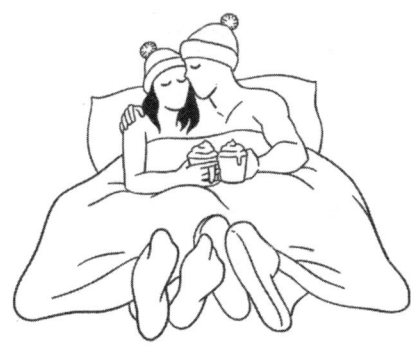

The Kettle Rating Scale™

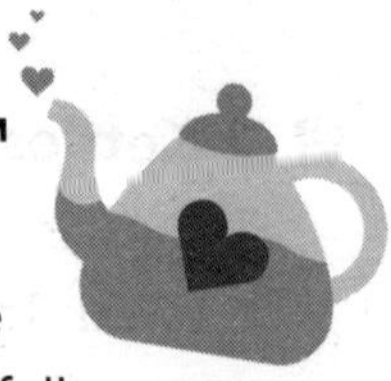

Not all cosy encounters are created equal – some are a gentle steep in tepid water, others are a full-blown boil on the hob of desire. Use our Kettle Rating Scale to track the heat of each position or act in this book, so you can select the one that's right for your mood – from 'just warming the pot' to 'call the letting agent, we've just warped the counter tops'.

1 Kettle – Lukewarm lovemaking

You've flicked the switch or turned the knob (the kettle metaphor depends on the type of appliance in your kitchen) and something's happening, but the water is still tepid. It's all gentle eye contact, soft touches and a lot of blankets. There's likely minimal movement but maximum snuggling. You might fall asleep halfway through – and that's okay.

2 Kettles – Warmed-up and willing

You've turned up the heat a little – there's a hint of curling steam but no risk of fogged-up windows just yet. You're warm… but not hot. Socks are still on. Biscuits might be involved.

♥ 3 Kettles – Simmering saucily

Things are steeping and decidedly getting brewed. These positions will definitely require some effort but the number of cushions will keep things measured and meaningful. You are officially glowing.

♥ 4 Kettles – Rolling-boil romance

Hot hot hot! Steam is being emitted and the kettle is whistling! Expect sweat – consider changing those flannel pjs for something a little lighter – and be careful! These positions involve lovemaking of such energy that you might accidentally knock over your mug.

♥ 5 Kettles – Too hot to sip

The kettle is as close to boiling over as the positions in this book get! The temperature's not unsafe for handling (try the original *Kama Sutra* if you want acts that require a metaphorical fire alarm), but you're going to have to remove the extra throw blanket for this – and socks are decidedly optional by this point.

Getting Started: Cosy Lovemaking Essentials

Equipment

To access the full range of positions in this book, you will need:

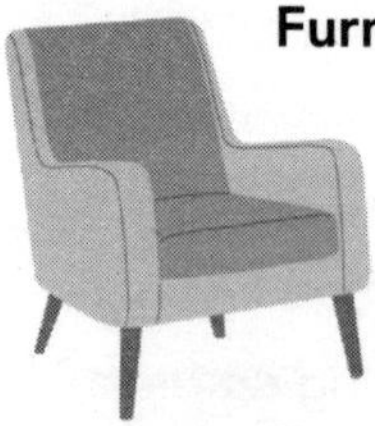

Furniture: sofa, Barcalounger (preferred) or armchair, straight-backed chair, fireplace with roaring blaze (or search 'relaxing crackling fire' on YouTube), bathtub.

Setting the scene: scented candles (chocolate, pine, forest cabin variously recommended), laundry detergent with washing machine, bubble bath, scent of gravy.

Soft furnishings: cushions, pillows, blankets, duvet, a weighted blanket, soft fabrics for draping, throws.

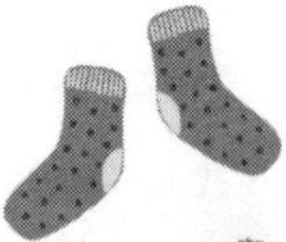

Clothing accessories: comfy bathrobe, slippers, thick socks, mittens, a very oversized jumper, flannel pjs, snood, woolly hat.

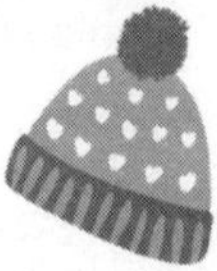

Edible goodies: chocolates (individually wrapped and bars for melting), your favourite baked goods, jam, a plate of spaghetti and meatballs, fondue pot with dippable goodies, icing, marshmallows, biscuits, apple pie with vanilla soft-serve ice cream.

Hot drinks: Earl Grey, chamomile tea, hot chocolate.

Games: Scrabble, Twister.

Accoutrements: breakfast tray, titillating feathers, warm teabag, saucy poetry books, craft materials to make a seasonal wreath (eucalyptus, pine cones, miniature pumpkins, twine, cinnamon sticks), a very, very large pumpkin, pumpkin-spice-flavoured lube, massage oils (cinnamon recommended), yoga mat.

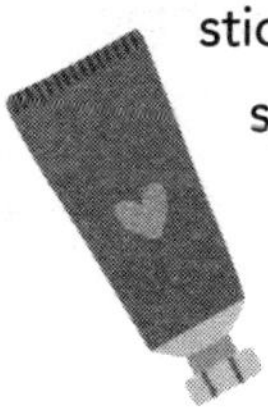

Aftercare and wind down

While many of the lovemaking acts in this book are already one big, luxurious wind down, if your romp was three kettles or above on the **Kettle Rating Scale™**, you'll want to bring yourselves gently back to a safe, lukewarm temperature. Think of this as the *cool-down stretch* of intimacy, but with more carbs.

Consider:

- **A warm towel wipe down** of any nude, sticky or chocolate-coated areas before re-donning clothes or pjs. A ritual that will leave both your soul and body cleansed.
- **Sharing a steaming mug** of tea, mulled wine or hot chocolate with extra marshmallows under the duvet – hydration and hygge.

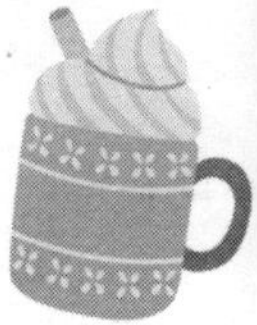

- **At least ten minutes of pillow talk**, preferably about completely inconsequential things ('Which *Bake Off* contestant do you think you'd be?').
- **Re-snuggling under the blankets** until you can no longer tell where one person ends and the other begins.

- **Cosy background TV** – *Gilmore Girls, Downton Abbey, The Holiday* – something comforting that won't kill the mood.
- **Post-sex snack plates** – cinnamon rolls, toast soldiers or whatever carbs your body is suddenly screaming for.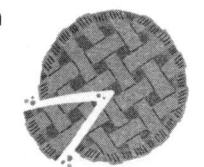
- **Synchronised nap**, also known as 'co-hibernation'.

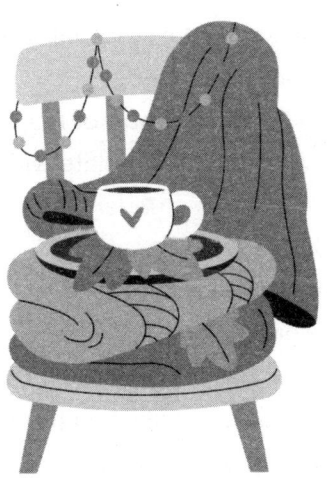

Sexy cosy foreplay playlist
Sittin' On My Sofa – The Kinks
Autumn Sweater – Yo La Tengo
we fell in love in october – girl in red
Mittens – Frank Turner
Sunday in Bed – Fluvny
Paws – Cashmere Cat
I Melt With You – Nouvelle Vague
Sleep Forever – Portugal. The Man
Let My Love Be Your Pillow – Ronnie Milsap
Autumn Leaves – Eva Cassidy
I Want a Little Sugar in My Bowl – Nina Simone
Night Moves – Bob Seger
These Arms of Mine – Otis Redding
Orinoco Flow - Enya

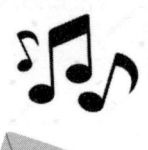

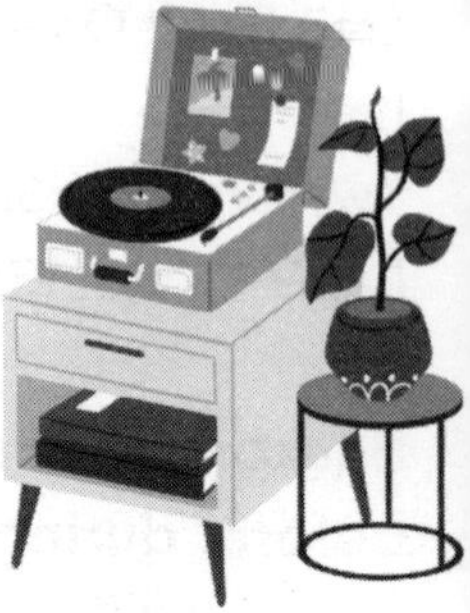

Getting down to it playlist
Turn Me On – Norah Jones
Earned It – The Weeknd
Fade Into You – Mazzy Star
Je t'aime... Moi Non Plus – Serge Gainsbourg and Jane Birkin
Love Serenade Part 1 – Barry White
Love to Love You Baby – Donna Summer

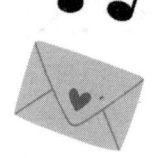

Let's Get It On – Marvin Gaye
I'm On Fire – Bruce Springsteen
By Your Side – Sade
L-O-V-E – Nat King Cole

Background calming sexy sounds for before, during or after

Rain sounds
Ambient cowbells
Purring noises
Ocean noises
Crackling fire
Soup simmering
Clinking radiator pipes
Knitting needles clacking
Washer on a spin cycle
Cats knocking things off shelves

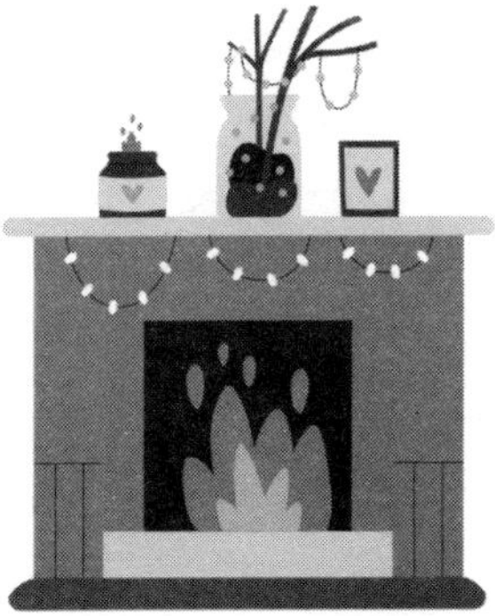

1

The Cinnamon Roll
(or *Kanelsnegle*, in Danish)

The receiver is on their front, curled up in a tight ball with legs tucked comfortably underneath them and their rear in the air. The giver massages their back with a thick layer of cinnamon-scented oil, then acts as the outer layer of pastry by draping themselves over the top of the rolled-up partner to enter them from behind (any flakiness in the outer partner is entirely optional but not recommended).

2
The 69-er

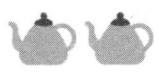

The couple slowly and sensually unwrap 69 little chocolates, then eat them while staring at each other lovingly. As 69 is an odd number, whoever gets the final chocolate performs oral sex on the other partner, as is only fair.

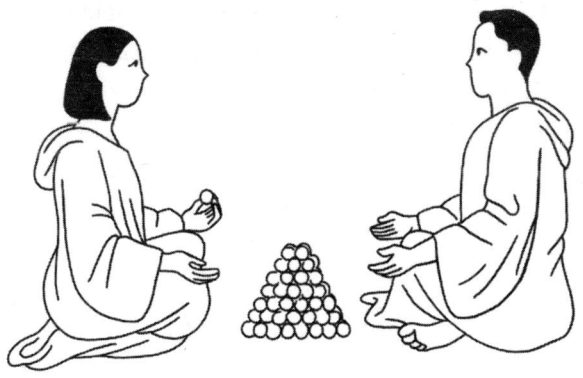

3

The Hot Choco-lotus

In this position, partners should imagine themselves to be marshmallows in a big, steaming cup of cocoa. To create the illusion, run a warm bath and light a chocolate-scented candle. Partners should then strip off and enter the bath quickly before experiencing any chill, then spend a few minutes enjoying the comfortable sensations of warmth and chocolate and happiness. Then they should either attempt to have sex – missionary position likely the easiest – or get out and finish with a cup of the real stuff.

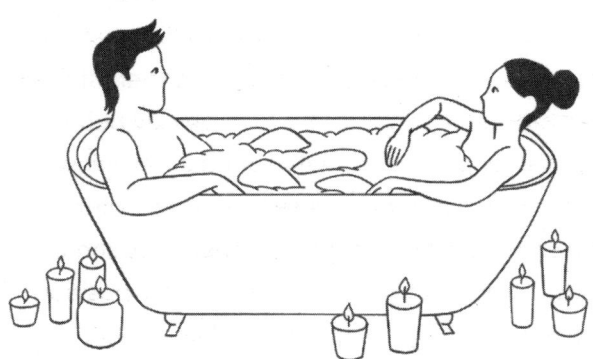

4

Robe Me the Right Way

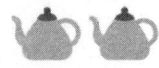

Two bathrobes, four wandering hands, zero chance of staying swaddled. Both partners should don their favourite comfy robe and lie down facing one another. Begin with gentle, exploratory touches through the fabric – a thigh graze here, a nipple brush there – before giving each other's belts a teasing tug and nudging those robes ever-so-slightly ajar. This is not a race to nakedness, it's a gentle excavation of pleasure as you discover the secrets under that fleecy exterior. And when you finally take things to the next level and pull your bodies together, keep the robes on.

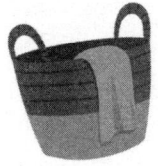

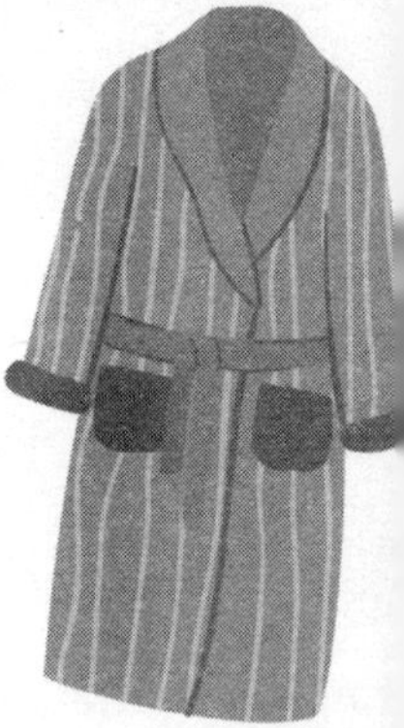

5

The Candle Canoodle

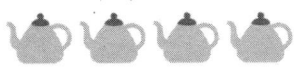

Surround yourselves with soft, flickering lights and throws. The giver sits cross-legged, leaning back a little so their lap imitates a candle holder. The receiver should perch on top of them, tall and proud like your favourite taper, then gyrate with quick, unpredictable movements like a flickering candle. You'll find yourself melting in no time as things heat up, but try not to make a mess, as wax is notoriously hard to clean up.

6

The Lazy Love Seat

Sometimes the idea of getting all worked up and finding props is just too much hard work and the cosiest thing you can think of is a quickie before dinner on the sofa. This position enables the least amount of time and effort, with the giver simply remaining seated on the sofa (the only action needed is to pull down their pants) and the receiver snuffling over to sit on top of them. You should consider pausing or at least muting the TV at this point. With a little mutual stimulation and a generous amount of lube, the receiver should slot on quickly and ride their partner's shaft to climax – before shifting back over to press play.

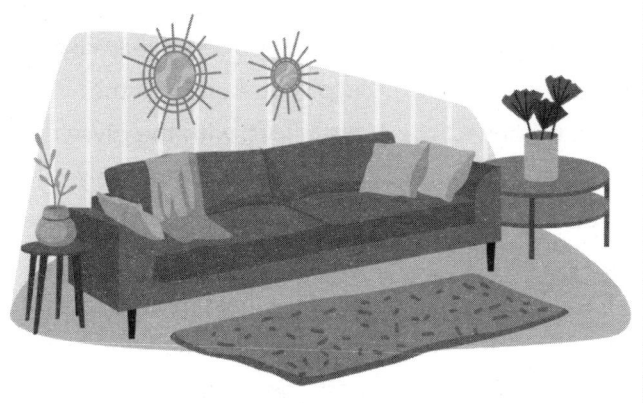

7

Sofa So Good

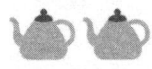

Want to make 'The Lazy Love Seat' even lazier? In this position, the giver lays back across the couch, propped up by at least three unnecessarily decorative cushions, legs draped over the armrest like a sexy croissant. The receiver remains straddling them, but this position allows for even deeper penetration and thus even less movement.

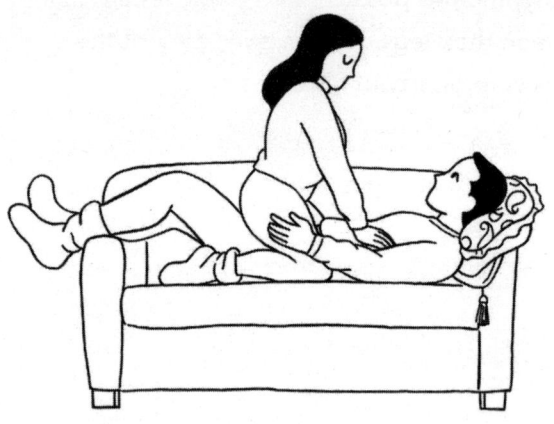

8

The Head Rush

Another position that doesn't require either partner to get up off the sofa, the giver positions themselves so their legs rest over the back of the sofa with their head and shoulders on the floor, resting on a soft pillow. As before, their partner rides them lazily, but in this position the blood will rush to the giver's head – both of them – creating mind-blowing orgasms. Alternatively, the receiver can assume this position with the giver crouched between their legs. Head rushes are not the exclusive property of either party.

9

The Danish Dip

There's something irresistibly snug about fondue. A bubbling pot at the centre of the table of warm cheese or chocolate, inviting slow, shared dipping, long forks crossing paths like old friends. No one rushes fondue. It's the meal equivalent of wearing a thick-knit jumper and having nowhere to be. It warms your hands, your belly and maybe – if things go the right way – your loins. In this position, there is no real fondue pot (see number 32 for the option). Instead, one partner lies on their back with their mouth wide open to simulate the fondue pot, while the other dips whatever body part they choose into it, lovingly.

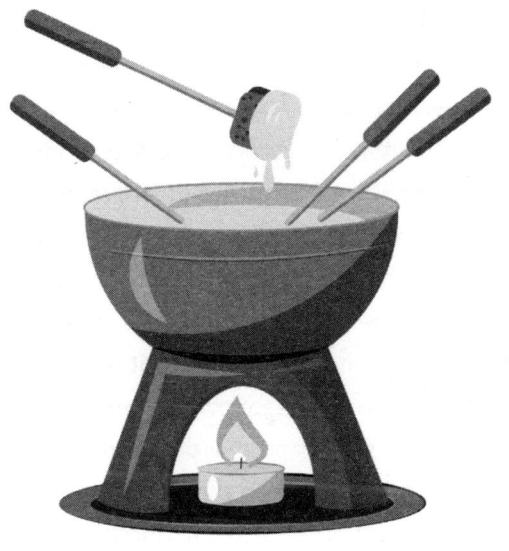

10

Knead Me Softly

Before things are ready to rise to the occasion in baking, sometimes a little preheating is needed – think a steady 150°C/300°F/Gas mark 2. This position can either be used as a warm-up before you try one of the other positions in this book, or maybe it's enough for you on its own. You've got nothing to prove (another baking pun, in case you missed it). To get started, lie your partner face-down on the bed and start kneading their tired muscles like a baker working dough, while speaking aloud all the innuendos you learned from *Bake Off*. Turn them onto their front to continue – if things are simply half-baked you might want to kiss and turn out the light. But if your partner is feeling the heat, it might be time to turn it up even higher.

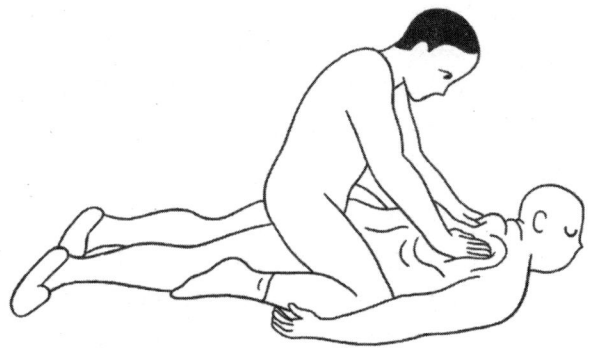

11

Roll Play

A sure-fire way to refresh things that have started to go stale in the bedroom is with some bread-themed roleplay. Combining sexual adventure with carbs will get things firing on all cylinders. Perhaps one of you is a high-powered city worker, who returns to their small home town when their family's bakery is in trouble? The other, a hungry local divorcee in desperate need of some sourdough to raise them out of their slump. You meet, you clash, you exchange some barbed jibes with an undercurrent of sexual tension, then make love on the kitchen table surrounded by baked goods and flour.

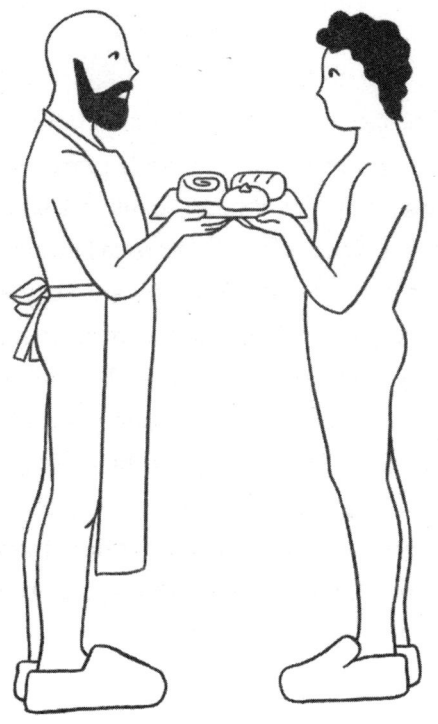

12

Tied and Toasty

Think BDSM, if the acronym stood for 'blankets, duvets, scarves and mittens'. One partner is blindfolded – cashmere only, thank you – and their wrists gently secured to the bedposts using soft scarves or knitted ties (we're going for restraint, not rope burn). Once comfortably secured, the other partner becomes a sensual sherpa of cosiness, using only gentle items (soft gloves, faux-fur hot water bottles) to tease and please. Think less *50 Shades*, more 50 Tog. The goal? To overwhelm them with so much warmth and anticipation that they practically melt, like a marshmallow on a radiator.

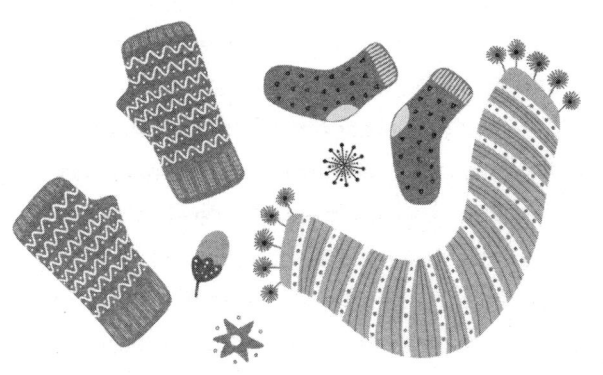

13

The Log Burner

Crouch by the fireplace (or search 'relaxing crackling fire' on YouTube if you don't have the real thing), while turning the radiators up a few notches. Partners should assume the classic 'doggy' position, with the receiver on all fours and the giver kneeling behind them. Because who is cosier than a dog by the fire? (Unless it's a cat, but that's not an argument that's worth having when you're this relaxed.)

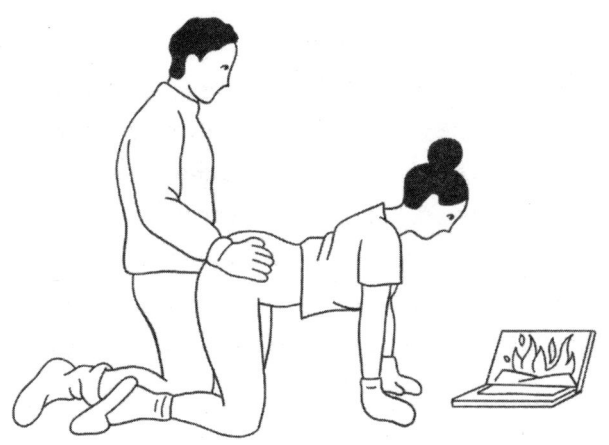

14

The Almost-nap

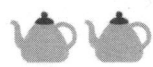

The giver lies flat on their back in what appears to be a peaceful doze – apart from one very awake appendage. The receiver mounts in reverse cowgirl, then reclines fully back, their spine flush to their partner's chest, legs stretched out and relaxed. It's lazy. It's languid. It's like having sex while pretending you're not. A slow, subtle grind can unlock some truly impressive sensations, especially if you choose to subcontract some of the effort to a vibrator (or some encouraging dirty talk). No sweat, no acrobatics – just good vibes and excellent lumbar alignment.

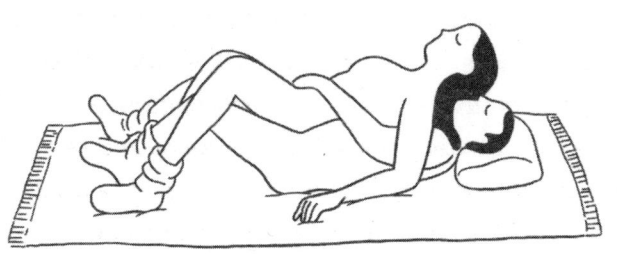

15

The Stomach-sleeper

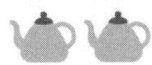

The receiver lies on their stomach with their head resting on their arms, as if they've already drifted off, their legs spread a little and a pillow placed under their pelvis. The giver lays their body over the receiver's and enters from behind – but instead of thrusting, moves in a circular, swirling motion. It's the sex equivalent of snoozing through a Sunday morning: all warmth and weight and barely-there effort. The giver can explore their partner's neck and back with their lips, tongue and teeth.

16
The 'Slip'

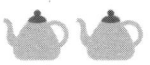

The receiver lies on their back, a soft pillow cradling their head, legs raised gracefully like a well-loved footrest. Slippers remain firmly on: this is not a drill. The giver kneels between those slippered feet and enters slowly, sensually. The mission? Maintain full penetration and slipper retention. This isn't just mindful sex, it's an act of balance, focus and foot-based affection. Eye contact: encouraged. Sock coordination: optional. Warm feet, warm hearts, satisfied everything.

17

The Blanket Statement

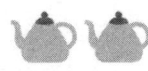

Outdoor sex isn't usually the go-to for hygge lovers – nature is beautiful, but so is central heating. However, with the right prep, *al fresco* can become al snugglo. First, scout a secluded, soft patch – think mossy nook or tucked-away garden corner – and lay down a thick, blanket base layer. Add a pillow (or two, you're not animals), then crawl under at least two more blankets like you're building a love nest. Once bundled together, find each other's *soft, sheltered spots* and proceed gently.

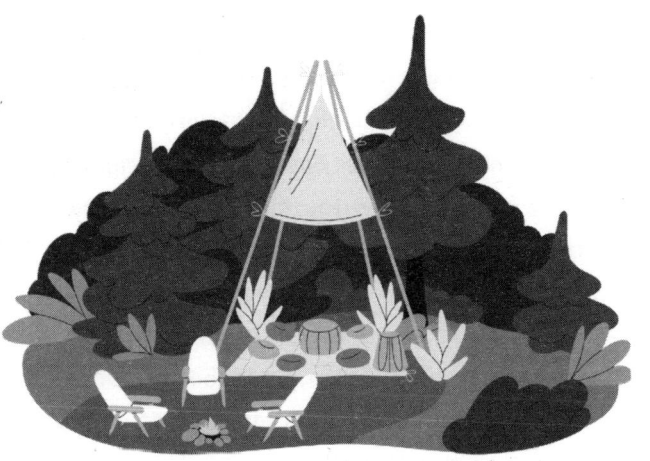

18

The Journal Entry

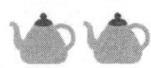

Gratitude journalling is known to boost happiness, reduce stress and improve sleep – but who says it has to be a solo activity? For a full-body dose of good vibes, lay your partner out on the bed like your favourite hardback. Check they're warm, comfy and ready to receive some very personal affirmations. Then open them up like a journal and prepare to make today's entry – the type that doesn't need proofreading. List all the parts of them you're most grateful for – out loud – and give each one a slow, reverential kiss. (Yes, *especially* that one. And that one too.) But be warned: while traditional gratitude journalling winds you down for bed, this version will have the opposite effect.

LOVE STORY

19

The Full Scone

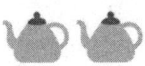

A British twist on the Danish bakes elsewhere in this book, this comes with a warning: things could get a bit sticky. It's the ultimate teatime indulgence and pairs beautifully with a cup of Earl Grey. One partner sits comfortably like a warm, freshly baked scone, while the other lovingly spreads jam on them. Slowly licking, savouring and savouring again, this position invites tactile teasing and is entirely delicious. Whether you end up adding the cream on top depends on how things progress.

20

Hygge Me Hard

Set an alarm for five minutes. Partners stand and face one another, enveloping each other in a tight embrace. Neither partner is allowed to move a muscle until the alarm goes off – well, some muscles may move involuntarily – but they should take it in turns to tell each other what they wish to do to their partner once the time is up. The temptation is to break the bear hug and start acting on those wishes, but this one is all about the delayed gratification.

21

Slip 'n' Slide

Start your day the steamy way with this wintry standing quickie, performed while both of you are wrapped in plush dressing gowns and wearing thick socks. No need to disrobe – just let those robes hang open like a seductive advent calendar. Choose your location wisely: the kitchen is classic (toast popping, coffee brewing – do you take cream with yours?), but take care on slippery floors. Nothing said 'mood killer' like an unexpected hamstring injury, but a little slipping and sliding can make for fun, unpredictable angles.

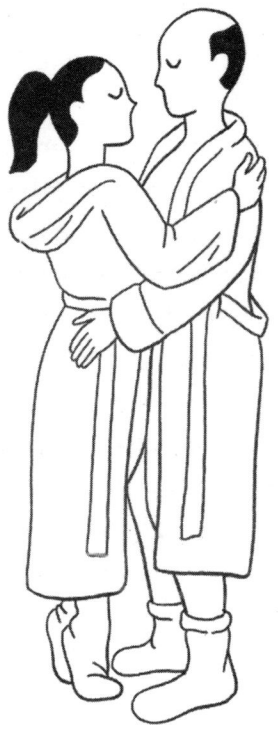

22

The 'Blow Me'

Slip into a warm bubble bath brimming with frothy clouds and scented bubbles, surrounded by candles. One partner lounges luxuriously, covered by suds, while the other leans in close to blow soft, teasing bursts of air across their skin, dispelling the bubbles and igniting goosebumps. This should be done without touching but with plenty of titillating. You can take it in turns and decide whether to stay in the bath long past the moment when you start to prune, or whether you want to move things onto the mat.

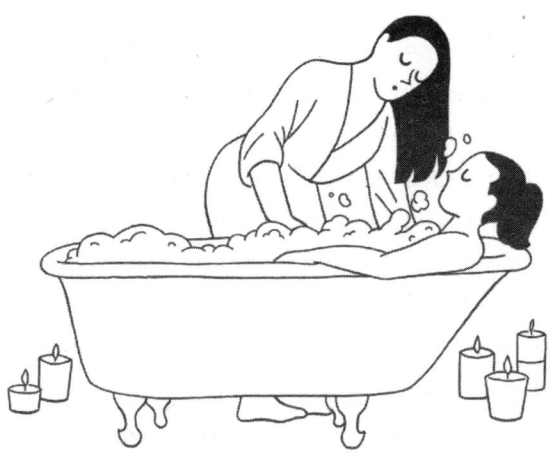

23

Paw Play

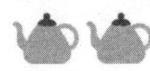

Both partners pull on soft mittens for a mutual manual adventure. Whether you start off naked or want to attempt undressing each other wearing your mitts (buttons can be a challenge) is your choice, but sometimes putting in the effort is the best way of showing you care. What you lose in dexterity you can more than make up for with enthusiasm. Proceed to paw at one another like overexcited woodland creatures on heat – nuzzling, softly biting and stimulating one another with your mitts. Fingering is, for obvious reasons, entirely off the table. But blunt-force fondling? Absolutely encouraged. Note: mittens will need to be washed before re-use.

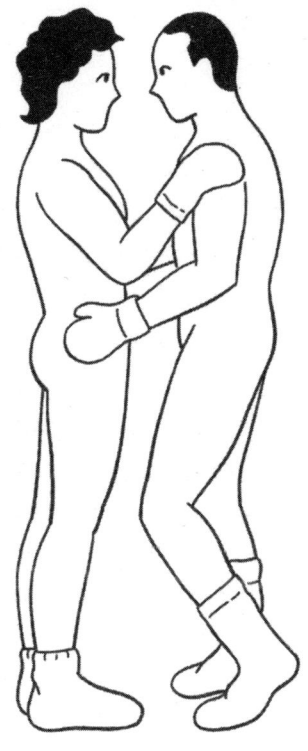

24

The Grotto Grope

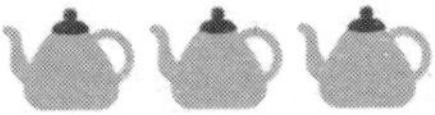

What could be cosier than transforming your bedroom into a magical grotto? String up fairy lights, drape soft fabrics over lamps and scatter pillows and blankets like a woodland nymph's nesting ground. It's all about the sensory experience, so consider pine-scented candles – or even forage for some of the real things on a trip to the woods. Once your enchanted love nest is ready, lie down and entwine limbs like the roots of an old oak tree; moans echo better in enchanted spaces. And if you climax under a canopy of twinkling lights while someone's antler headband falls off? That's not weird, that's being *committed to the theme*.

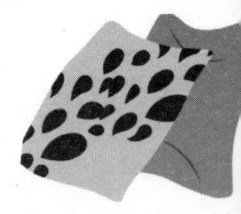

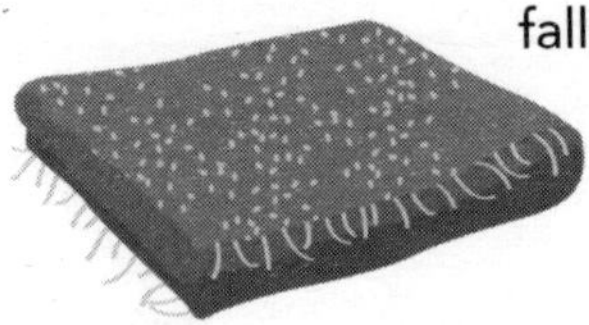

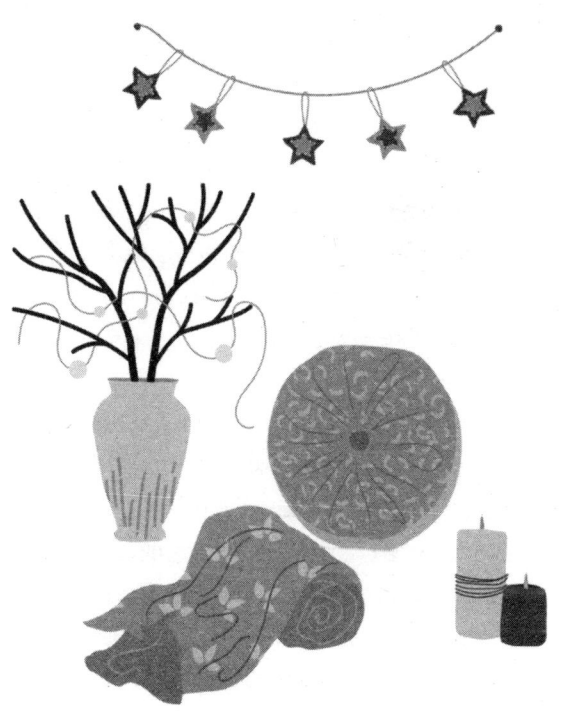

25

Worth the Weight

You'll need to get yourself a weighted blanket for this one – but think of the purchase as an investment in your mental health and your pelvic floor. These magical adult swaddles are known to reduce anxiety, promote sleep and, as it turns out, deliver the perfect conditions for slow-motion spooning sex. One partner lies behind the other, both tucked under the heavy, comforting embrace of 10kg of blanket that says, 'You're not going anywhere fast, and that's a good thing.' With all frantic thrusting options kindly removed by gravity, you're left with one choice: deep, purposeful, inch-by-inch intimacy. It's languid. It's luxurious. It's a bit like shagging in slo-mo while wearing a hug. And, hey, if you fall asleep mid-thrust, that's not a failure, it's therapeutic.

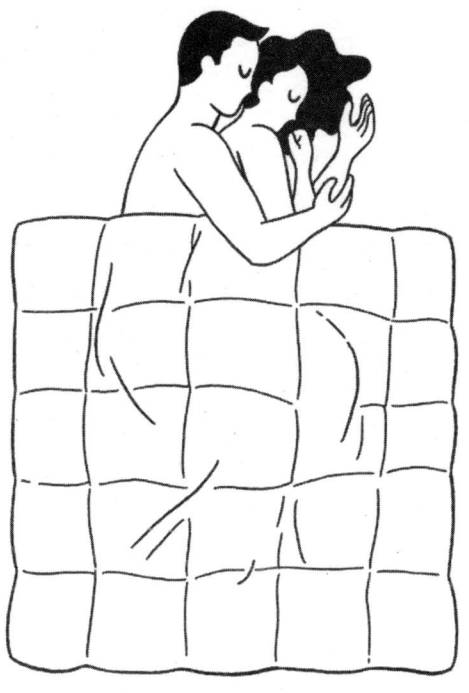

26

The Mixing Spoon

A variation on the classic spoon, where a receiver with a clitoris will find that the introduction of a battery-powered tool really mixes things up – rather like how an electric stand mixer would supercharge your baking. Partners should assume the spoon position, but this time the receiver should raise their top leg and tuck it behind their partner's. The receiver, while making sweet love to the giver from behind, reaches around to pleasure their partner with a vibrator. It will really stir things up.

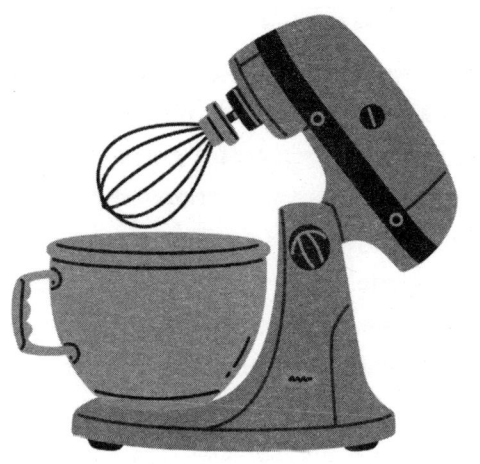

27

The Spaghett-about-it

There's a special level of comfort that is reached after an Italian dinner – the doughy, drowsy magic that only a generous helping of carbs can bring. And what could deliver that better than a *Lady and the Tramp*-inspired foreplay session: slurping spaghetti while making eyes at each other or popping meatballs (veggie option available) suggestively into your mouths? It is imperative that you re-enact the famous meet-in-the-middle moment from the film faithfully, for full romance. Then, when you are quite full, passionately fling everything off the table and build on the feeling of mutual satisfaction with some classic on-the-table missionary.

Note: tomato sauce stains are hard to get out, so continuing the intimacy with a shared bleaching of the tablecloth in the bath afterwards is recommended.

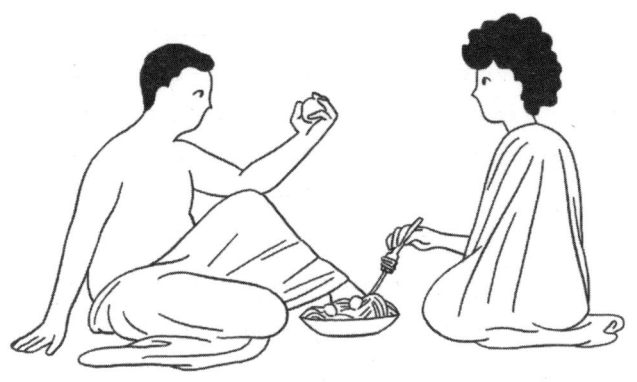

28

The Spin Cycle

For many, one of the most comforting smells is that of fresh laundry – whether it's something floral or more earthy, like sandalwood. If you're lucky enough to have a laundry room, it can be a veritable playground of pleasure, but all you really need is a washing machine. Simply assume the position of 'The Lazy Love Seat' (see number 6) while perched on top of the machine on its highest spin setting, and the combination of the motion, steady 'white-noise-' style sound and luxurious aroma will have your mind relaxed and your body opening up to
the centrifugal force.

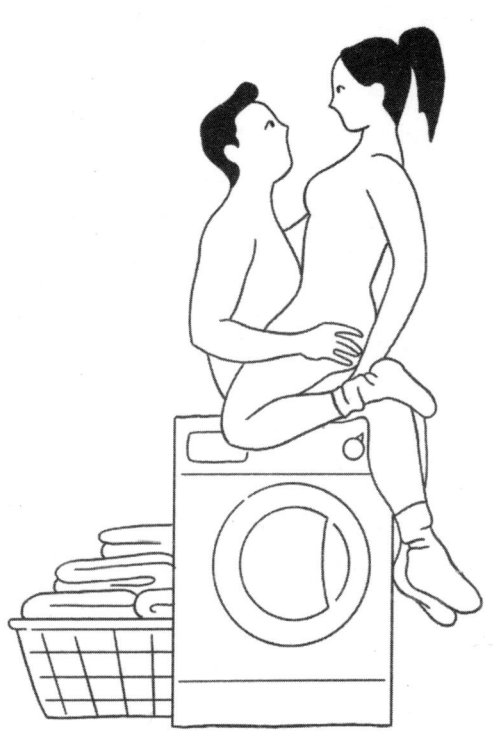

29

Clean Is the New Dirty

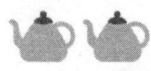

Take the love for that fresh laundry smell and feel to the next level – lay clothes fresh from the dryer on the floor, and make love missionary-style on their fragrant warmth. Depending on the scent, you'll be transported straight to the forest floor, beach or meadow.

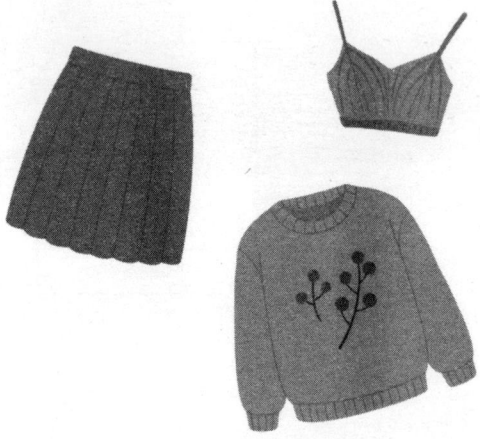

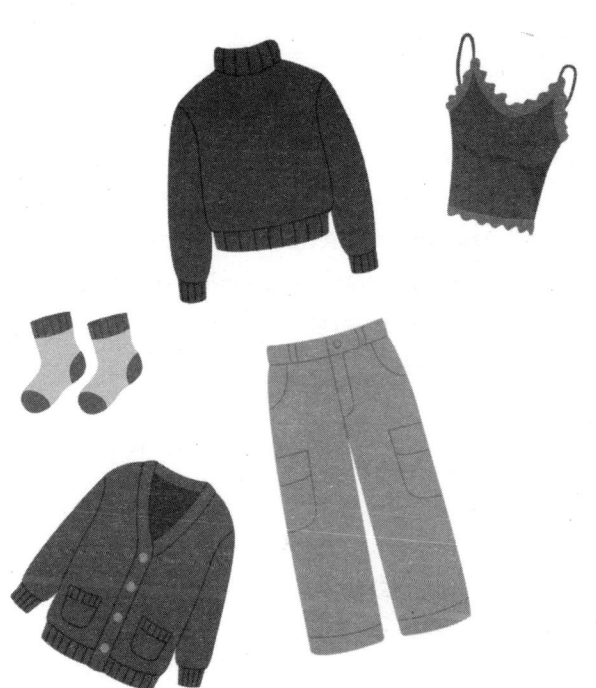

30

Wool You Be Mine

This one requires some pre-prep and skills with the old knitting needles – or a game grandma to help you out. You'll need to knit or have knitted a massive jumper, so large that you and your partner can both fit inside it, faced towards each other. When you're ready, get into position inside the knitwear with the receiver straddling their partner, naturally pressed together by the constraints of the garment. Slowly, testing the give of the material, start riding as one. This position is guaranteed to make you hot in more ways than one.

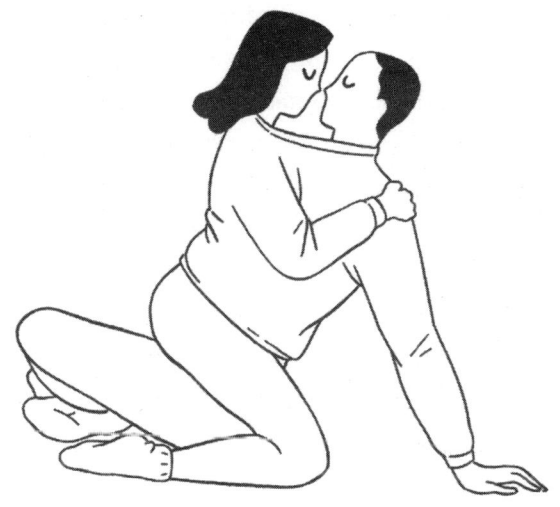

31

La-Z-Boy

Inspired by *Friends*, the comfort watch of a generation, this one's for those who like their sex with maximum chill and minimal core engagement. The giver settles into a Barcalounger-style sprawl (on an armchair, sofa or even propped up on too many pillows), assuming the sacred position of 'person who is absolutely not getting up anytime soon'. The receiver climbs aboard, facing away, then gracefully slumps backwards until they're resting like a human blanket across their partner's chest. Who moves depends on who had carbs at dinner, but it's all about slow thrusting or lazy grinding. Perhaps you'll whisper something like, 'Could you pass the remote?' No cardio, no pressure, but aim to finish before the Netflix 'Are you still watching?' message appears, otherwise inertia may set in.

32

The Fondue You

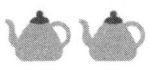

Position yourselves comfortably around a fondue pot filled with melted chocolate and an array of dippable goodies. Take it in turns to spear and dip said goodies, feeding them to each other romantically, before dipping your own less-edible but still delicious goodies for your partner to lick chocolate off. Double-dipping is not only allowed, it's encouraged.

33

The Rocking Chair

You may have thought this delightful piece of furniture was somewhere far into the glorious future for you, but you needn't wait until blissful retirement – you can simulate it now! The giver (ideally in a supportive, cushioned, high-backed chair) spreads their legs like they're settling in for a quiet evening and a Werther's Original. The receiver sits down on the giver, facing them, then – with the giver holding their elbows to keep them from falling – leans all the way backwards, legs up on their partner's shoulders like a flexible pension fund. And the resulting rhythm? Deep, slow and soothing – as if you were both swaying in a seaside hammock after your final mortgage payment.

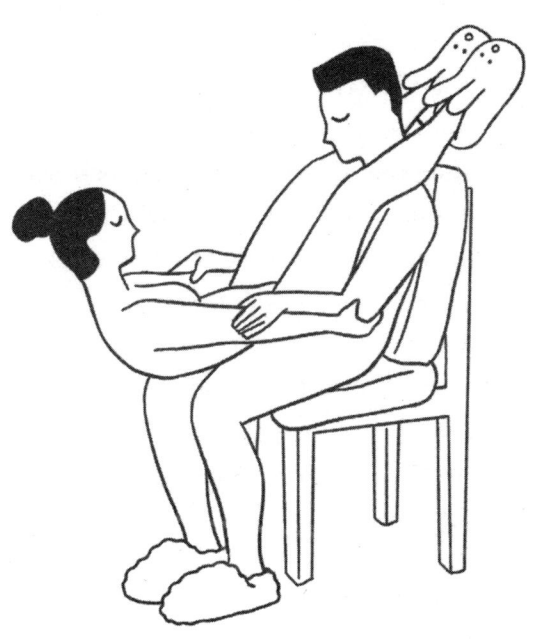

34

Strip Scrabble

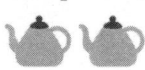

Settle by the fire with your favourite word-based board game, wearing plenty of clothing, and put on some sensual classical music (this is a classy game, after all). Proceed to play as per the standard rules, but every time your score reaches a multiple of 50, the other player must remove an item of clothing. Whoever is the last player wearing any clothes is the winner and their prize is to receive oral sex on top of the Scrabble board (you may wish to remove the tiles first).

35

Saucy Scrabble

Because one filthy version of the world's cosiest game could never be enough! In this version, players must aim to spell out body parts with their tiles – LABIA, TOE, ANUS, BREAST, PENIS – then choose whether it's their own body part or their partner's that is to be stimulated. The player chosen must then arouse their partner by licking, sucking or biting that body part for thirty seconds. You still score as in the traditional game, but you can decide whether the real winner gets the most points or ends the game with the most sexual pleasure.

Note: for added sauciness, remember that Scrabble is a 2–4-person game.

BREAST
TOE
PENIS
LABIA
ANUS
SCRABBLE

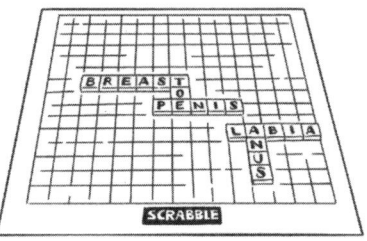

36

Tantric Twister

Another game you can play in the comfort of your own home. Just make sure you crank the heating up for this one, as it's one of the few practices in this book that demands nudity – you'll even have to remove your socks, or you'll slip on the mat! Once naked, proceed to play Twister as per the usual rules, but if you have a free hand or foot and can reach, you should be using it to fondle your partner (just not so much that they fall down). If your spin brings your face close enough, you can even get your tongue involved.

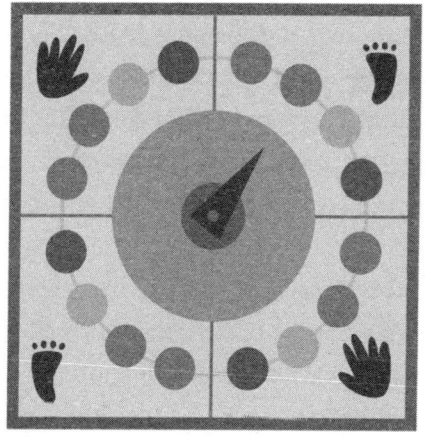

37

Sunday Roast

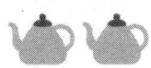

This super-cosy position isn't just reserved for Sundays — though it does pair beautifully with the scent of gravy in the air and a late-afternoon nap pending! The receiver lies curled up on their front, knees tucked under and rear lifted into the air, rather like a turkey ready to be stuffed. The giver kneels behind and does the stuffing, ideally with the kind of reverence normally reserved for heirloom Le Creuset cookware. Optional extras include a drizzle of massage (or sunflower) oil, a Yorkshire pudding cooling on the nightstand and the smell of rosemary in the air.

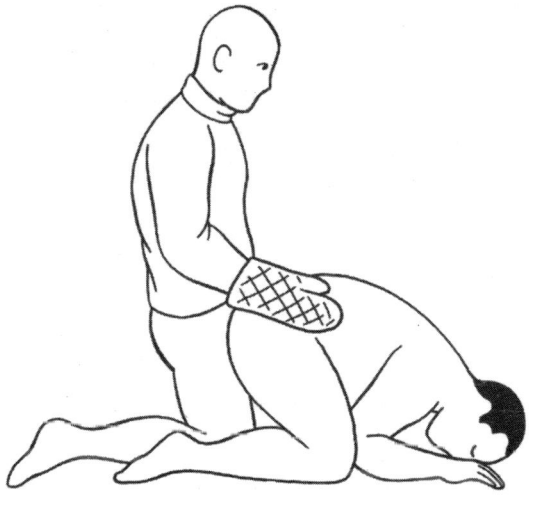

38

The Danish Pastry

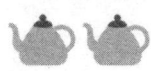

This sweet and sticky position is perfect for when you want closeness, eye contact and just the right amount of indulgent mess. Start by facing each other, both seated with legs wrapped around one another, pretzeled like the breakfast treat of your dreams. You should be skin to skin, hips aligned, arms around each other like you're about to slow-dance to a Sade song. Now for the pastry part: drizzle real icing across each other's shoulders, collarbones, or wherever your inner patisserie chef guides you. Then, take your time slowly licking it off as you begin to move together, gradually, like your bodies are sizing in a slow bake. And when you're both finally spent, you'll collapse into each other like buttery layers of pastry, possibly needing a flannel and a snack.

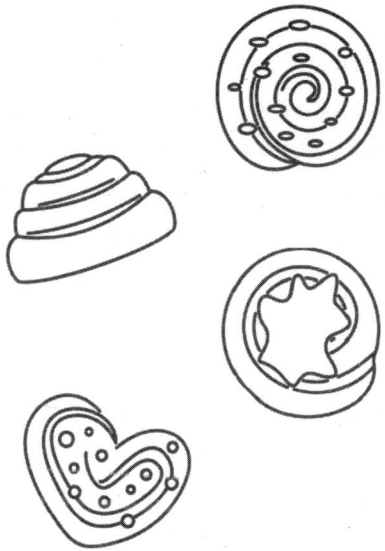

39

Feline Frisky

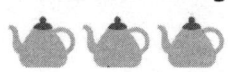

Who knows comfort better than a cat? For this position, get dressed in your softest threads, find a classic cat-friendly spot around the house (the end of the bed, a patch of carpet where the sun hits just right, or by a radiator) and the receiver should assume a sphinx-like pose on their knees, with forearms on the floor and bum in the air. The giver should make love to their partner from behind, leaning over them so their bodies are touching as much as possible, and nibbling their neck occasionally.

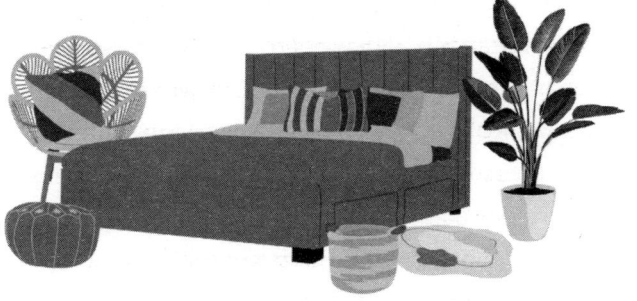

40

Lazy Dog

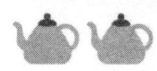

This is a bit like a collapsed version of the traditional 'doggy' position. The receiver lies on their stomach with arms bent at the elbows. Legs are splayed out, one knee bent lazily to the side, as if they might stretch or sigh but they never actually move. The giver lies on top, facing the receiver and matching this position, like a weighted blanket with intentions. Entry is from behind, but effort is minimal. Think of it less as thrusting and more as slow, sleepy rocking – like trying to gently soothe each other to orgasm while whispering 'Who's a good human?' into each other's ears. Where this takes place depends entirely on your pet policy. On the bed? Great. On the sofa? Cosier. On the floor with a dog watching you judgementally from their own blanket pile? That's between you and your therapist.

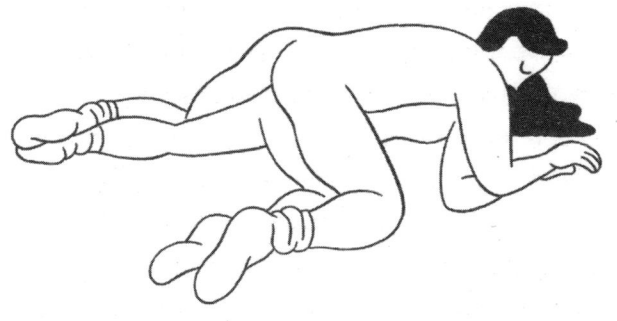

41

Breakfast in Bed

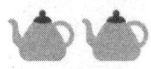

Because who says the toast is the only thing getting buttered? This is ideal for lazy mornings with nowhere to be. One partner plays the attentive lover: delivering a warm cup of tea, maybe a bit of toast – something light, because the real meal is coming next. Once the tray is set and appreciation expressed, it's time for the server to help themselves to a more personal kind of nourishment; ideally between the thighs, not between bites. Bonus points for keeping the mug steady during oral. It's intimate. It's indulgent. It's a full English, minus the baked beans and finishing with optional sausage.

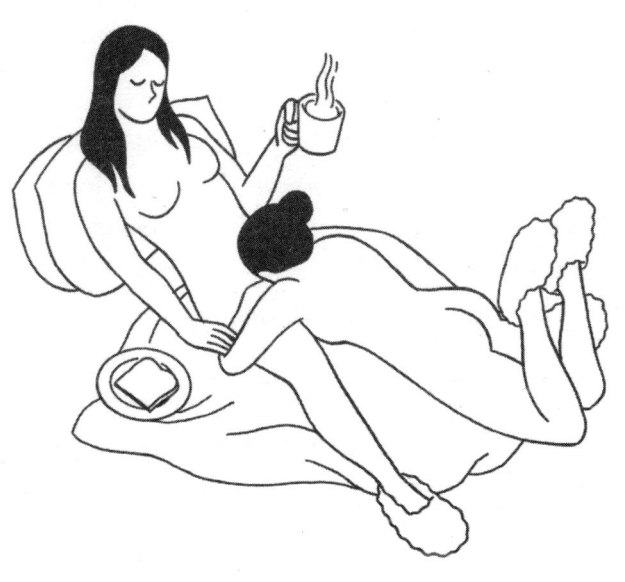

42

The Toast Rack

This works best with some friends. Line up as many as are present, all facing forwards like a line of little soldiers, so you're almost touching. Each lover reaches forward to fondle the person in front of them, while the person at the back, the oft-forgotten end-piece, must have the dual job of pleasuring themselves as well as the person in front. Every few minutes, the person at the front should peel off to stand at the back, while everyone else takes a step forwards.

43

Fancy a Nap

A bit like a traditional lap dance… except this low-effort, high-snuggle number involves the 'dancer' climbing into their partner's lap fully clothed – ideally in flannel pjs, fluffy socks and with a vaguely seductive yawn. The dancing should mainly consist of slowly swaying to a playlist of Enya songs or the gentle hum of a dishwasher, with the dancer's head gently nestled into the crook of their partner's neck. This position thrives in the sweet spot between foreplay and full-on hibernation. It could turn into more, or it could result in one of you snoozing, the other wondering if this still counts as sex. (It does.)

44

Robe One Out

The ultimate in slow, teasing undress – without ever actually undressing. The performer enters the room in a fluffy bathrobe and socks to begin the slowest, most suggestive reveal of individual body parts, while the rest stay toasty warm. You might bare a shoulder dramatically, then cover it up again quickly. Perhaps you'll part the robe to show a wayward nipple, then close it again. Maybe you'll slide a hand under the robe to describe what's underneath and how it's responding to your touch. All the while telling your partner, 'You don't get to see ankle until you've earned it.' The key is eye contact, confidence and commitment to the slow burn. End with a final, dramatic straddle or cuddle, wrapping the robe around both of you like a sultry towel burrito. If things escalate from there, great – if not, you still get to keep your robe and your dignity.

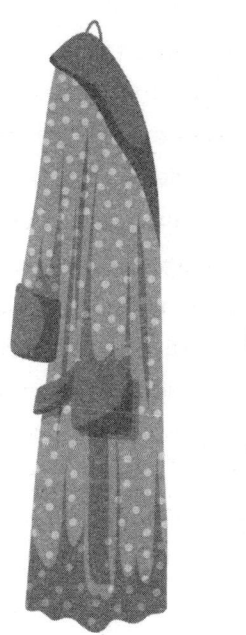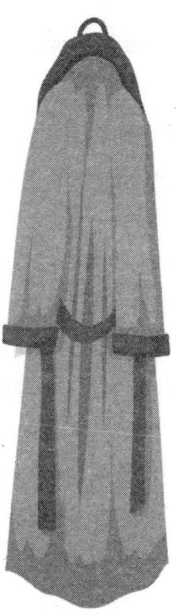

45

In the Snood

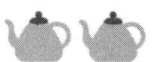

Grab your comfiest snood, soft enough to nuzzle but not so thick you'd struggle to breathe through it. One partner slips the snood over their neck and pulls it up just high enough to partially cover their mouth; think of it as a peekaboo balaclava. They then begin to kiss, lick or gently blow their partner through the soft fabric. The sensation is warm, fuzzy and delightfully filtered, like oral sex on the softest difficulty setting. Think of it as a sensual tease, a tickly prelude, like muffled devotion with a side of static cling.

46

The Slow Cooker

Set it and let things simmer. This position is all about low-and-slow sensuality, like a stew that takes all day but is so worth it. Both partners lie together in a tight cuddle, facing one another, whispering steamy nonsense in one another's ears like, 'You smell like sourdough' or 'I want to baste you.' The key is to build heat gently. Think warm breath on the neck, gentle thigh strokes, lingering kisses, all while keeping body contact continuous and pressure deliciously low. Movement is minimal. Every shift of a hip or roll of a shoulder should feel deliberate and languid, like melting butter. You're not racing to the finish, you're letting the flavour develop. This is ideal for lazy Sunday mornings, rainy evenings or any time you'd rather slow-roast your sex life than flash-fry it.

47

Do the Hygge-Boogie

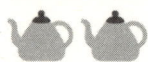

This one starts out innocently enough: just two people, dim lighting and some smooth jazz or mellow lo-fi beats. Arms go around necks. Hands rest gently on waists. You sway together like it's a school disco and someone's playing Norah Jones on a cassette tape. But here's the twist: you're not 11 anymore, and there's no teacher chaperoning. You can move in as close as you like: chests brushing, hips grinding, erogenous zones making contact like two magnets in fleecy pyjamas. The magic is in the build-up, with a shared rhythm, soft breathing, wandering hands. Keep dancing until one of you decides to slip a hand somewhere exploratory – or until someone gets dipped dramatically onto the bed like the end of a very raunchy rom-com.

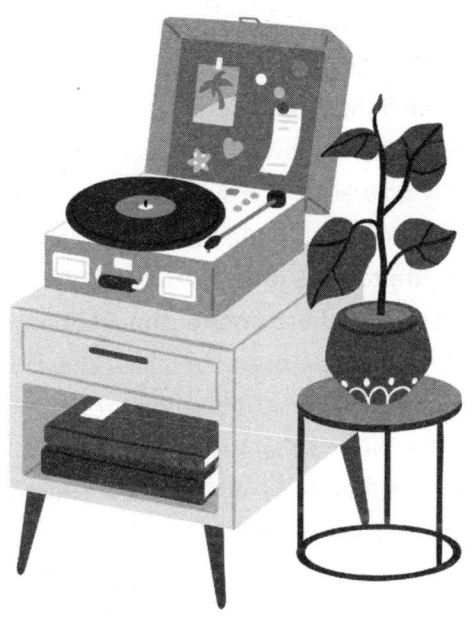

48

Soothe Operator

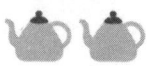

This is another one that slips more into the foreplay category, but an erotic hygge massage is less about deep tissue and so much more about fostering a deep sexual connection. Begin by setting the scene the hygge way: fairy lights glowing, slippers off and light a candle that smells like 'forest cabin'. One partner should lie face-down with a bare back, with a cosy blanket over their bottom half. The other should sit astride them, warm a little massage oil between their palms and begin a slow, intentional massage. Think less 'sports massage' and more 'butter melting on a warm croissant'. Long strokes.

Circular motions. Occasional detours towards pleasure zones that are definitely not in the wellness manual. Whisper sweet nothings like 'Your shoulders are so sexy when unclenched' or 'Is it hot in here or is it just your lumbar region?'

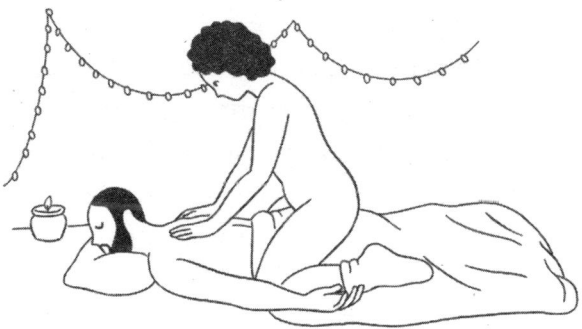

49

Pillow Tease

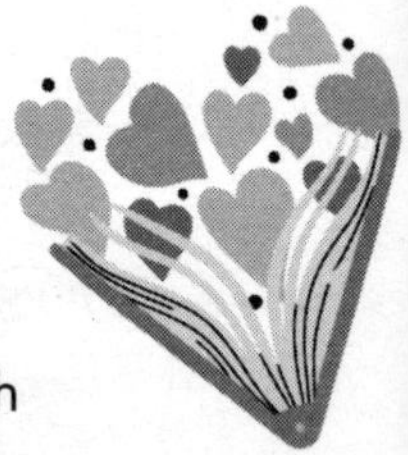

Lie facing each other under a shared duvet, legs just barely brushing, your faces close enough to feel each other's breath but with a firm no-touching rule in place. This one's all about verbal intimacy – a kind of hygge striptease for the soul. Take turns whispering sexy-but-soft things to each other, designed not just to get each other hot but to warm your souls, too. Think: 'I want to slow-roast you like a winter stew'; 'I want to unbutton your cardigan emotionally first' or 'You make me feel like a hot water bottle that's been held all night'. This is about building tension, not releasing it (yet).

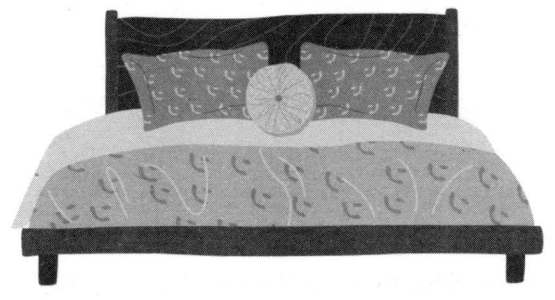

The key is to linger in the anticipation – the longer you can keep it going without touching, the more electric it becomes. By the time someone breaks the no-contact rule (and someone will), you'll both be primed for a very warm, very cosy explosion of affection.

50

Happy Baby Yoga

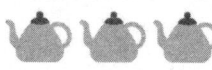

Yes, it's literally called Happy Baby, and it is a little awkward, but don't let that put you off! This classic yoga pose is about joyful surrender, gentle openness and letting it all go (tension, pants, inhibition). The receiver lies on their back, knees bent and pulled towards their chest, then reaches between their legs to grab their toes. This position isn't just adorable, it's practical: hips are open, access is excellent, and rocking side to side can be incredibly soothing. Meanwhile, the giver kneels, facing the business end. From there, they can gently enter wherever consensual exploration takes you – vaginal, anal or simply spiritual. The combination of eye contact and flexibility makes this pose both vulnerable and powerful.

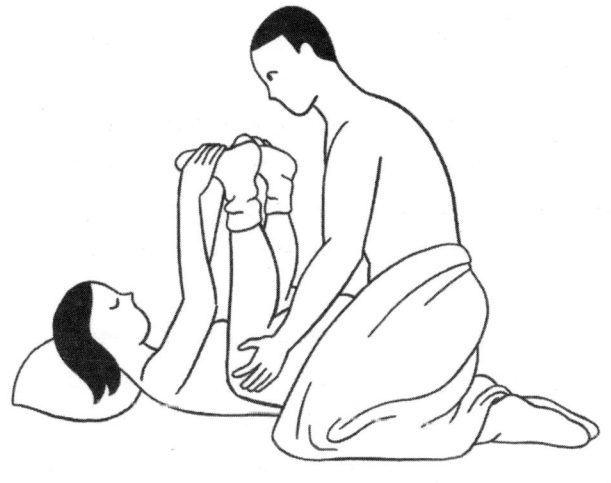

51

The Blanket Offering

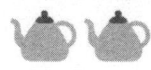

Child's pose is another unfortunately named yoga position, but get that association out of your head as this pose is definitely just for adults. It's all about devotion, surrender and putting your bum in the air in the most wholesome way possible. The receiver folds forward into this yoga pose with knees wide, arms outstretched or tucked under, forehead resting gently on the bed or floor. The giver spoons behind, applying slow, steady pressure, stroking along the spine, or slipping into a very gentle rocking rhythm and, when the receiver is ready, enters with strong, slow thrusts. A weighted blanket over both partners makes this even cosier.

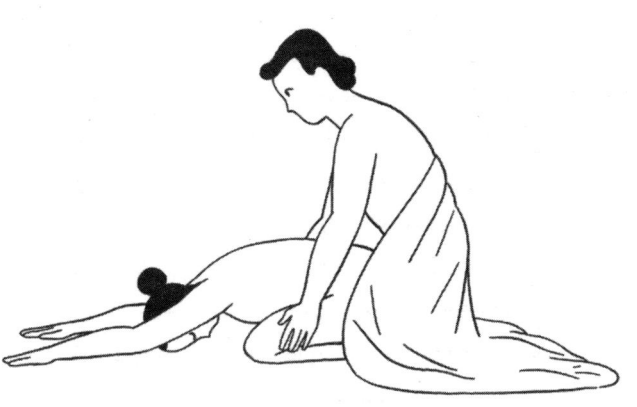

52

Purr and Moo

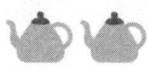

No, it's not a new Scandi crime drama, it's a sensual, synchronised grind utilising the yoga 'cat/cow' poses. Start on all fours, facing each other if you're feeling intimate, or one behind the other for a shared rhythm. Move slowly between arching and dipping your spine, inhaling and exhaling in time. This is less about penetration at this point, more about foreplay and flow. And when the time is right, the receiver should come to a perfect tabletop that you could balance your hot chocolate on, before the giver moves into position behind them. Optional soundtrack: ambient cowbells and gentle purring noises.

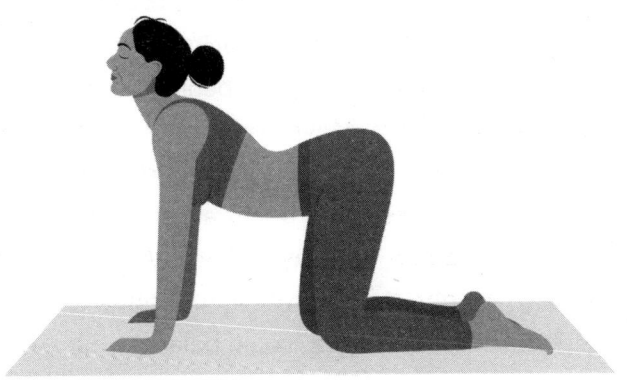

53

Pre-coital Savasana

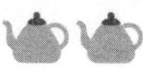

One partner, post a few yoga poses to loosen up the joints, lies on their back, limbs flopped open in *Savasana* (corpse pose). They should allow their minds to empty and all tension to leave their bodies. The other partner assembles an arsenal of toys to tickle, titillate and stimulate them, from soft feathers and fluffy socks to a warm teabag (squeezed first). This continues until the receiving partner can't take it anymore and wants to get back into a downward dog.

54

Post-coital Savasana

Arguably not an in-action sex position – but yes, I will argue with that actually, because who says sex stops straight after climax? Any good lover knows sensuality shouldn't stop the second you're done, as this is the perfect moment to foster true intimacy. So once you're finished and have completed any toilette, allow yourself to be warm, glowing logs of satisfaction among the glowing embers of your lovemaking. One of you lies flat on your back in corpse pose. The other might offer gentle words, soft caresses, or just lie next to you, equally corpse-like. Movement is strictly forbidden. Intimacy is not.

55

The Open Book

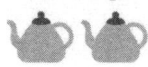

Lie back with the soles of your feet together, knees dropped out to the sides like a half-read romance novel – in the yoga pose *Supta Baddha Konasana* (butterfly pose). Tuck cushions under your thighs, neck and back. This position is excellent for oral sex, lazy fingering or gentle visual appreciation. If the vibe is right, one partner can straddle gently and read a poem aloud. Or just say filthy things in a soothing voice. It's a choose-your-own-adventure.

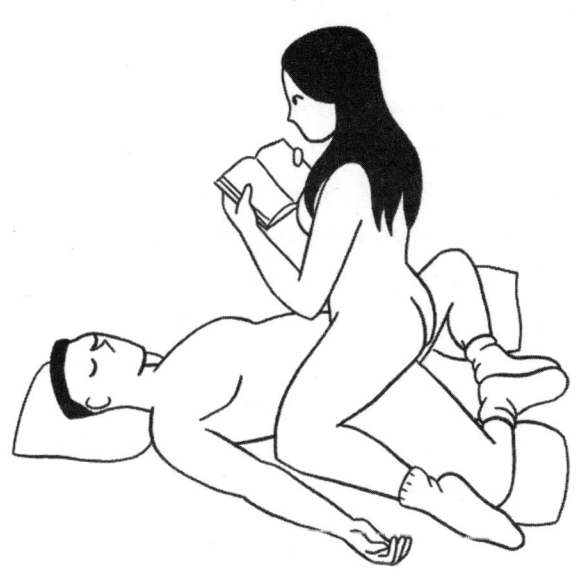

56

Putting Your Feet Up

This restorative yoga pose, known colloquially as 'legs up the wall', is ideal for end-of-day intimacy. Lie on your back with legs up against something solid, hips elevated with a cushion or firm pillow. Blood flows from your toes to your core. Your partner can sit beside you, stroke your thighs, nibble on your calves or just talk about their day while stroking your arm. If oral happens, it's the kind you sip slowly like a perfectly brewed tea. Recommended: chamomile.

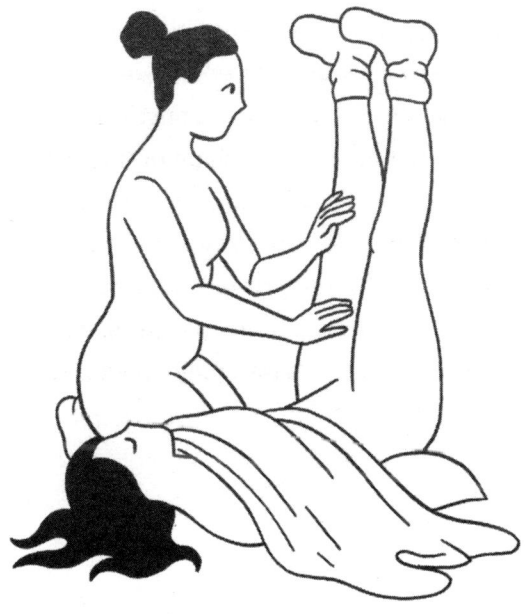

57

Log Cabin Heat

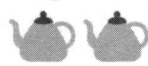

Settle in across from your partner, both of you cross-legged with shins stacked like logs in a woodburner – this yoga pose is, after all, known as 'fire log'. Bring your foreheads together like you're sharing a secret (or trying to charge each other like phones). Breathe in sync, hold hands and gently sway like you're generating friction-based intimacy. When you're thoroughly snuggled and spiritually aligned, keep those eyes closed and let your hands begin a slow and exploratory journey – over shoulders, waists, thighs and anywhere that makes your partner exhale like a kettle. The goal? To lovingly bring each other to climax without ever standing up. You're not just sitting, you're simmering. And like any good cabin weekend, there's no rush to leave.

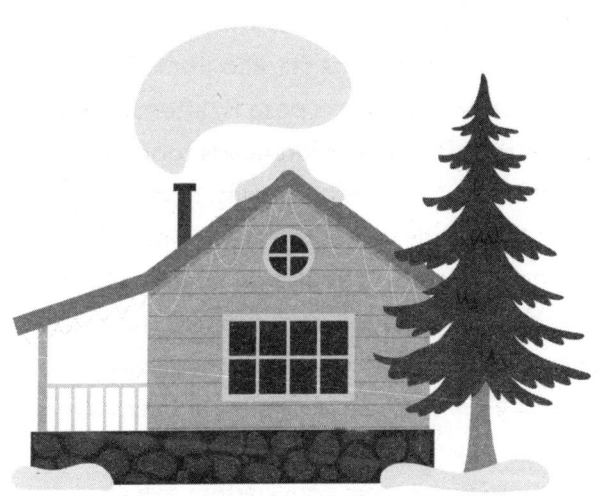

58

Give Me S'more

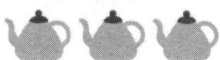

When you want something messy, melty and emotionally satisfying, skip straight to dessert. Start by assembling proper s'more ingredients: marshmallows, chocolate and biscuits. Toast marshmallows together, feeding them to each other slowly – yes, it's sticky, yes, it's messy, and yes, that's the point. Drizzle melted chocolate on a finger and offer it up for licking. Let the sweetness linger on your lips and trade kisses that taste like a sleepover fantasy gone very adult. When you're good and gooey, lie your partner down and make a 'human s'more': place a warm marshmallow on their chest or belly, a square of chocolate on top, and gently lick it off; slowly, sensually, with ridiculous reverence. The biscuits can crumble; your self-control already has. Then? Get horizontal. You're both already warm, melty and stuck together in the best possible way.

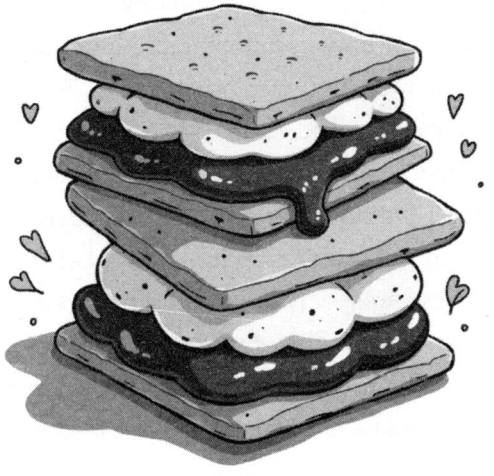

59

The 'Woman From Ealing'

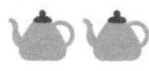

Poetry has long been used to stir hearts, loins and – in this case – whatever's within reach under the blanket. While battle epics might kill the mood (unless you're into horny *Iliad* roleplay), a sensual sonnet or smutty limerick can work wonders. Start simple: one partner reads aloud something flirtatiously filthy, such as Sappho, Shakespeare or something you found in an old *Cosmo*. Meanwhile, the listener caresses themselves or their partner in time with the rhythm. For a more interactive version, sit face-to-face and create your own erotic poem together, each attempting a rhyming couplet and acting out the naughty lines as you go. It's like foreplay, but with metaphor and metre.

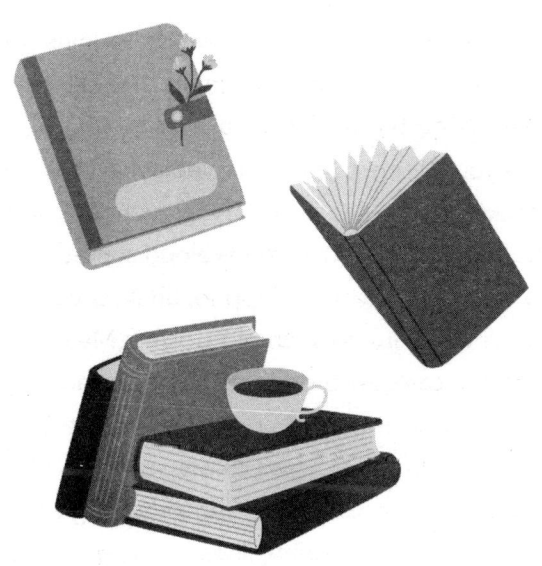

60

The Plough

No tractors involved – unless that's your thing – this move is named for the constellation. Stargazing is peak hygge for the Danes, especially when the Northern Lights are doing their thing. But if the skies aren't cooperating, this position will have you seeing stars regardless. The giver lies flat on their back while the receiver mounts them in a classic cowboy. From there, the receiver leans backwards with hands resting on their partner's knees, chest skyward, eyes on the heavens, spine gently arched. Its equal parts stretch and straddle, and great for slow, rhythmic movement. Ideal for a clear, warm night on a blanket under the stars – or just indoors with some stick-on glow-in-the-dark stickers on the ceiling. It's also calling for some great astronomical sex-talk: 'Uranus is looking great tonight', 'They call it the Big Dipper for a reason', 'I'm ready to get lost in your wormhole', etc.

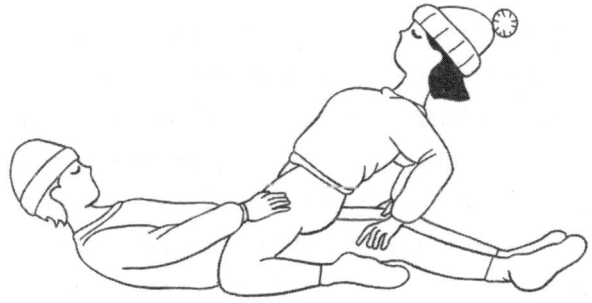

61

Guided Meditation

A session that starts with 'Ommm' and ends in 'Ohhhh yes.' One partner sits cross-legged on the floor, nude except for their socks (because cold feet are not cosy). The other, equally sock-clad and starkers, settles in behind them with their chest pressed warmly against their partner's back. Wrap a fluffy blanket around you both, if needed – think tantric burrito. The partner in the back takes the lead, guiding the other through a sensual meditation. Start with something soothing: 'You are alone in a quiet forest, birdsong in the distance, a soft breeze across your skin.' Then slowly raise the temperature: 'The breeze is my breath on your neck. The birdsong is my heartbeat. And can you feel… my wood?'

Begin to gently kiss, stroke or whisper them into blissful arousal. The goal is to calm, then arouse, then perhaps transcend both entirely. By the time you reach full-body nirvana, your chakras won't be the only thing that's aligned.

62

Wreathed in Pleasure

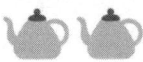

Like *Ghost*, but with pine cones. You and your partner begin an innocent-enough craft session: making a seasonal wreath for the front door. Think winter pine and eucalyptus, or autumn leaves and miniature pumpkins. One partner takes the lead on the crafting, sitting on a sturdy chair or low stool. The other settles in behind, arms wrapped lovingly around them, both contributing to the hot glue and holly action. Hands entwined, you guide each other in positioning sprigs just right, threading twine and occasionally accidentally brushing fingers or letting one hand linger a bit too long on a firm bauble. The scent of cinnamon sticks and forest foliage fills the room.

Eventually, it's less about the door décor and more about the front door access. Clothes may come off. The wire cutters stay safely aside. You finish each other and the wreath, which now holds far more sentimental value than anything store-bought.

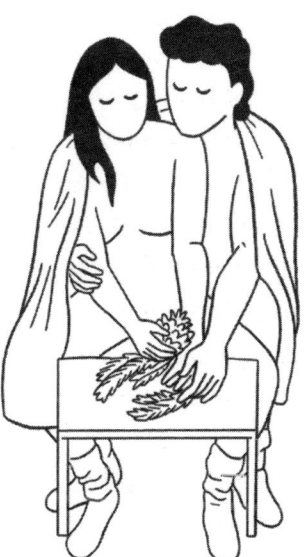

63

The Throw-down

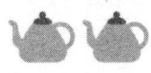

This may not be the dramatic, passionate sex you're imagining from the name. Rather, it's missionary, but you need to put a comfortable throw-down first. You can do it on the bed, on the sofa, on the floor – just make sure it's a throw that's machine washable and soft, and you're ready to go.

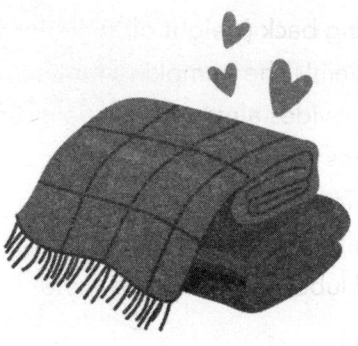

64

Pumpkin Spice

No scent quite says autumn-cosy like pumpkin spice – in this position, you'll be using a pumpkin to spice things up in the bedroom. First, source a large pumpkin – ideally selecting your own from a pumpkin patch with your partner, frolicking in the fields as you anticipate the use you'll be putting your gourd to later. Once home, the receiver should remove their many layers of knitwear to sit astride the pumpkin, opening their legs wide and leaning back (weight on their arms or a sofa behind them). The pumpkin's firm, rounded surface provides a natural, gentle incline that encourages a slow, rocking motion. The giver kneels in front of them proceeds to give them oral – ideally after firstly applying some pumpkin spice-flavoured lube (yes, it is a real thing).

65

Harvest Season

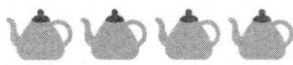

Embrace autumn with this wheelbarrow-simulated position. The receiver kneels on a cushioned stool with their hands placed on the ground – ideally resting on a folded blanket for comfort.
The giver enters the receiver, using their legs or hips as leverage to control the rate and depth of thrusting. This position is perfect after a day of apple-picking to get you both in the mood.

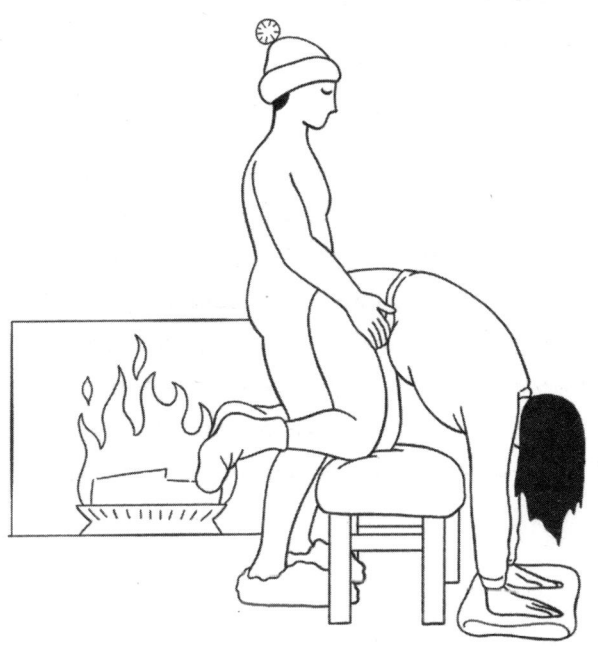

66

Pulling the Wool Over Your Eyes

For this sexy game, you will need a sexy woolly hat, ideally with a bobble on top. The seeker dons the hat, pulling it down low over their eyes, effectively turning it into a snug and stylish blindfold. The other player must be almost entirely naked (socks are, as ever, optional) and dabs a generous amount of melted chocolate on one area of their body. They then lie down in front of the seeker, who must use all their senses to locate the chocolate and lick it off. You can continue to play, taking turns, until the chocolate sets or you're hungry for more.

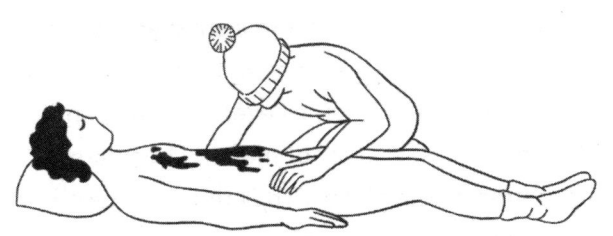

67

The Facial Treatment

The ultimate cosy night in surely has to involve some sort of pampering – how about this twist on a classic face mask? In this act, one partner lies prone on the bed in a comfortable position, but instead of placing a sheet mask over their visage, the other partner should position themselves so they're seated over the giver's face. The giver should then proceed to give their partner slow and meaningful oral.

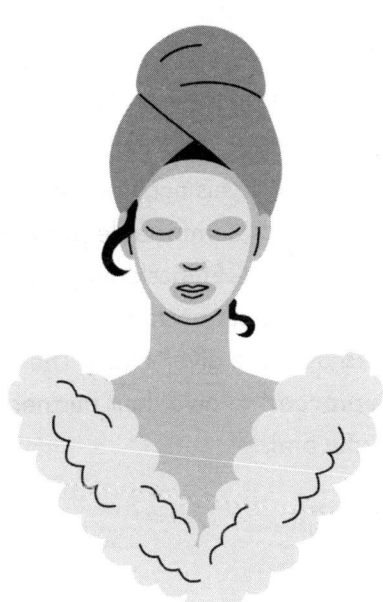

68

Cute As Apple Pie

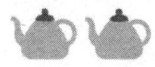

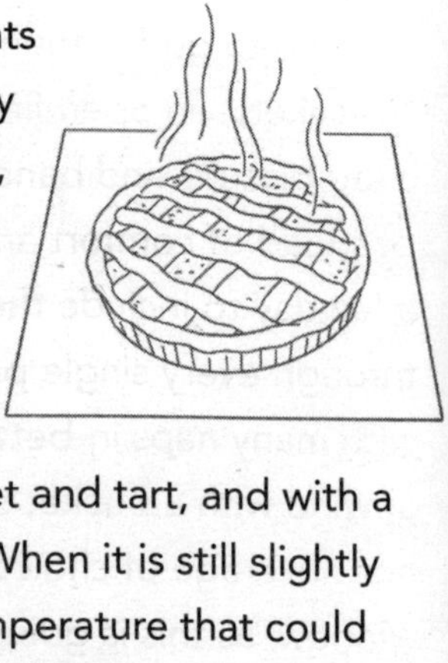

To remind you of movie nights of yore, this act is inspired by the classic film *American Pie*, and is perfect for a seasonal treat. First, you will need to bake a delicious apple pie, with a filling that is the perfect combination of sweet and tart, and with a thin, faintly crispy topping. When it is still slightly warm but certainly not a temperature that could scald, you can take it in turn to dip body parts into the pie, then allow your partner to lick off the sweet dessert. If you want to play with different sensations, you could also introduce a scoop of vanilla soft-serve ice cream.

69

The Full Hygge

It's time to go full theme. Everything's involved – blankets, an open fire, candles, knitwear, body heat, biscuits and banging. A total sensory overload of comfort and carnality. Allow at least a full day to include the slow warm up, to work through every single position or act in this book with many naps in-between, then it's time to unwind with a bucket-sized cup containing your hot beverage of choice. And make sure to crack a window, as this is going to get too steamy to be truly comfortable, and the last thing you want to do is overheat.

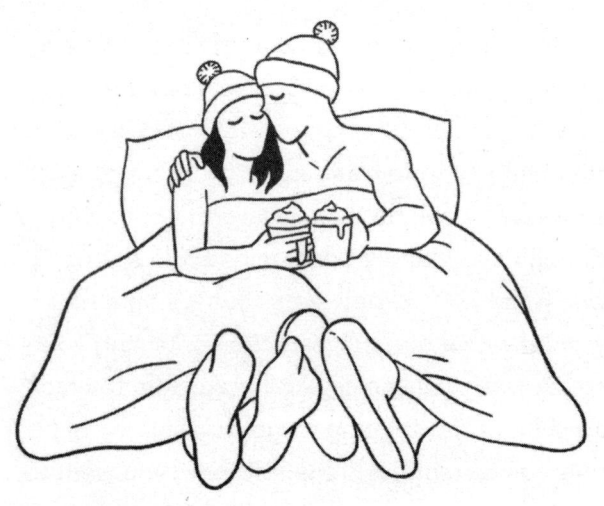